CONTENTS

INTRODUCTION

Introduction to "The Acid Reflux Cookbook: Delicious and Reflux-Friendly Recipes for Better Digestion"

Acid reflux, also known as gastroesophageal reflux disease (GERD), affects millions of people worldwide. It's a condition that occurs when the stomach acid flows back into the esophagus, causing discomfort and irritation. While medication can help manage symptoms, dietary changes are often the first line of defense in reducing the frequency and severity of acid reflux.

That's where "The Acid Reflux Cookbook" comes in. This cookbook is designed to provide delicious and reflux-friendly recipes for better digestion. Whether you're a seasoned cook or a beginner in the kitchen, you'll find a range of options to suit your taste preferences and dietary needs.

In this cookbook, you'll learn about the foods and ingredients that can trigger acid reflux and the ones that can soothe and prevent symptoms. You'll also find practical tips and techniques for cooking that are gentle on the stomach, as well as guidance on how to make reflux-friendly choices when dining out.

But most importantly, you'll find an array of delicious recipes that are low in acid, gentle on the stomach, and packed with flavor. From breakfast to dinner, snacks to desserts, and even drinks and smoothies, there's something for every meal and occasion.

The recipes in this cookbook are not only reflux-friendly,

but they're also healthy and nutritious. You'll find a variety of options for vegetarian, meat-eaters, and fish lovers, as well as for those who prefer sweet or savory dishes.

In addition to the recipes, this cookbook also includes a range of resources to help you on your journey to managing acid reflux. You'll find information on the different types of acid reflux and their symptoms, as well as advice on lifestyle modifications and stress management techniques that can help reduce symptoms.

We hope that "The Acid Reflux Cookbook" will be a valuable resource for those who suffer from acid reflux, as well as for their families and loved ones. With these delicious and reflux-friendly recipes, you can enjoy a varied and satisfying diet while managing your symptoms and improving your quality of life.

CHAPTER ONE

Introduction To Acid Reflux And Its Symptoms:

Acid reflux, also known as gastroesophageal reflux disease (GERD), is a condition in which the stomach acid flows back into the esophagus. The esophagus is a tube that connects the mouth to the stomach, and it is not designed to handle the acidic contents of the stomach. When the stomach acid flows back into the esophagus, it causes irritation and inflammation, leading to a range of uncomfortable symptoms.

Acid reflux is a common condition that affects millions of people around the world. It can occur at any age, but it is more common in adults. The condition is caused by a weak lower esophageal sphincter (LES), which is a ring of muscle that separates the stomach from the esophagus. When the LES is weak, it allows the stomach acid to flow back into the esophagus, causing acid reflux.

Symptoms of Acid Reflux

The most common symptom of acid reflux is heartburn, which is a burning sensation in the chest. This sensation may be accompanied by a bitter or sour taste in the mouth. Other symptoms of acid reflux include:

- Regurgitation: This is when the stomach acid flows back into the mouth or throat. It may cause a sour or bitter taste in the mouth, and it can be accompanied by a feeling of nausea.

- Difficulty Swallowing: Acid reflux can cause difficulty swallowing, as the esophagus may become inflamed or narrowed.
- Chest Pain: Acid reflux can cause chest pain, which may be mistaken for a heart attack. The pain may be sharp or burning and may worsen after eating.
- Sore Throat: Acid reflux can cause a sore throat, especially in the morning. The throat may feel dry or scratchy, and there may be a hoarse or raspy voice.
- Chronic Cough: Acid reflux can cause a chronic cough, which may be worse at night or early in the morning. The cough may be dry or accompanied by mucus.
- Asthma: Acid reflux can worsen asthma symptoms, such as coughing and wheezing.
- Dental Problems: Acid reflux can cause dental problems, such as erosion of the enamel and tooth decay.

Effects of Acid Reflux on the Body

Acid reflux can have a range of effects on the body. When the stomach acid flows back into the esophagus, it can cause inflammation and irritation. Over time, this can lead to the development of a condition called Barrett's esophagus, which is a precancerous condition that increases the risk of esophageal cancer.

Acid reflux can also cause a range of respiratory problems, such as asthma and pneumonia. When the stomach acid flows into the lungs, it can cause inflammation and irritation, leading to breathing difficulties. Acid reflux can also worsen existing respiratory conditions, such as chronic obstructive pulmonary disease (COPD).

Acid reflux can also have an impact on dental health. The acid can erode the enamel on the teeth, leading to tooth decay and other dental problems. Acid reflux can also cause bad breath and a sour taste in the mouth.

Treatment of Acid Reflux

- The treatment of acid reflux depends on the severity of the condition and the symptoms. Mild cases of acid reflux can often be treated with lifestyle changes, such as:
- Diet: Avoiding spicy, fatty, and acidic foods can help reduce the symptoms of acid reflux. Eating smaller meals and avoiding large meals before bedtime can also help.
- Weight Loss: Losing weight can help reduce the symptoms of acid reflux, as excess weight can put pressure on the stomach and LES.
- Elevating the Head: Sleeping with the head elevated can help prevent the stomach acid from flowing back into the esophagus.
- Avoiding Alcohol and Tobacco: Both alcohol and tobacco can weaken the LES and increase the risk of acid reflux.

In more severe cases, medication may be necessary to manage the symptoms of acid reflux. There are several types of medications that can be used, including:

- Antacids: These are over-the-counter medications that neutralize the acid in the stomach. They can provide immediate relief from the symptoms of acid reflux.
- H2 Blockers: These are medications that reduce

the amount of acid produced by the stomach. They can be taken as needed or on a regular basis.

- Proton Pump Inhibitors (PPIs): These are medications that block the production of acid in the stomach. They are often prescribed for people with more severe cases of acid reflux.
- Prokinetics: These are medications that help the stomach empty more quickly, reducing the amount of time that the acid stays in the stomach.

In some cases, surgery may be necessary to treat acid reflux. Surgery is usually reserved for people with severe cases of acid reflux who have not responded to other treatments.

In conclusion, acid reflux is a common condition that can cause a range of uncomfortable symptoms. It occurs when the stomach acid flows back into the esophagus due to a weak LES. Symptoms of acid reflux include heartburn, regurgitation, difficulty swallowing, chest pain, sore throat, chronic cough, asthma, and dental problems. Acid reflux can have a range of effects on the body, including inflammation, irritation, and the development of precancerous conditions. The treatment of acid reflux depends on the severity of the condition and the symptoms, and may include lifestyle changes, medication, or surgery. If you experience symptoms of acid reflux, it is important to speak with your doctor to determine the best course of treatment.

Understanding The Causes Of Acid Reflux:

Acid reflux is a common condition that occurs when the contents of the stomach flow back up into the esophagus, causing uncomfortable symptoms such as heartburn, regurgitation, and chest pain. While occasional acid reflux is normal, frequent or chronic acid reflux can be a sign of an underlying medical condition. In this chapter, we will discuss the various causes of acid reflux, including lifestyle choices, diet, and medical conditions.

Lifestyle Choices:

Certain lifestyle choices can increase the risk of acid reflux. These include:

- Being overweight or obese: Excess weight can put pressure on the stomach and cause the contents to flow back up into the esophagus.
- Smoking: Smoking weakens the lower esophageal sphincter (LES), making it easier for stomach acid to flow back up into the esophagus.
- Drinking alcohol: Alcohol can also weaken the LES, making it easier for stomach acid to flow back up into the esophagus.
- Eating large meals: Eating large meals can increase the pressure in the stomach and cause the contents to flow back up into the esophagus.
- Eating before bedtime: Eating before bedtime can also increase the risk of acid reflux, as lying down can make it easier for stomach acid to flow back up into the esophagus.

Diet:

Certain foods can trigger acid reflux by increasing the production of stomach acid or by weakening the LES. Some of the foods that can trigger acid reflux include:

- Spicy foods: Spicy foods can increase the production of stomach acid, making it more likely to flow back up into the esophagus.

- Acidic foods: Foods that are high in acidity, such as citrus fruits and tomatoes, can also trigger acid reflux by irritating the lining of the esophagus.
- Fatty foods: Fatty foods can weaken the LES, making it easier for stomach acid to flow back up into the esophagus.
- Chocolate: Chocolate contains caffeine and theobromine, which can relax the LES and increase the risk of acid reflux.
- Carbonated beverages: Carbonated beverages can increase the pressure in the stomach and cause the contents to flow back up into the esophagus.

Medical Conditions:

There are several medical conditions that can increase the risk of acid reflux. These include:

- Hiatal hernia: A hiatal hernia occurs when part of the stomach pushes through the diaphragm and into the chest. This can weaken the LES and increase the risk of acid reflux.
- Pregnancy: Pregnancy can increase the pressure on the stomach, making it easier for the contents to flow back up into the esophagus.
- Scleroderma: Scleroderma is a rare autoimmune disorder that can affect the connective tissue in the body. This can cause the LES to weaken and increase the risk of acid reflux.
- Gastroparesis: Gastroparesis is a condition in which the stomach takes longer than normal to empty its contents. This can increase the risk of acid reflux by allowing the contents to stay in the stomach for a longer period of time.

- Eosinophilic Esophagitis: Eosinophilic Esophagitis (EoE) is a chronic allergic inflammatory condition of the esophagus that can cause acid reflux-like symptoms.

Medications:

Certain medications can increase the risk of acid reflux by relaxing the LES or by irritating the lining of the esophagus. Some of the medications that can increase the risk of acid reflux include:

- Calcium channel blockers: Calcium channel blockers are medications used to treat high blood pressure. They can relax the LES and increase the risk of acid reflux.
- Antidepressants: Antidepressants can also relax the LES and increase the risk of acid reflux.
- Bisphosphonates: Bisphosphonates are medications used to treat osteoporosis. They can irritate the lining of the esophagus and increase the risk of acid reflux.
- Nonsteroidal anti-inflammatory drugs (NSAIDs): NSAIDs can irritate the lining of the esophagus and increase the risk of acid reflux.
- Potassium supplements: Potassium supplements can irritate the lining of the esophagus and increase the risk of acid reflux.

In conclusion, acid reflux is a common condition that can be triggered by a variety of factors. Lifestyle choices such as being overweight, smoking, and drinking alcohol can increase the risk of acid reflux. Certain foods such as spicy foods, acidic foods, and fatty foods can also trigger acid reflux. Medical conditions such as hiatal hernia, pregnancy, and scleroderma can increase the risk of acid reflux. Finally, certain medications such as calcium channel blockers, antidepressants, and bisphosphonates can also increase the risk of acid reflux. By understanding the causes of acid reflux, individuals can take steps to reduce their risk and manage their symptoms.

The Acid Reflux Diet:

Acid reflux, also known as gastroesophageal reflux disease (GERD), is a condition that affects millions of people worldwide. It occurs when the stomach acid flows back up into the esophagus, causing discomfort, pain, and sometimes even damage. While there are several medical treatments for acid reflux, making dietary changes can also help alleviate the symptoms. In this chapter, we will focus on the acid reflux diet, outlining the foods to avoid and the ones to include in a reflux-friendly diet.

Foods to Avoid

Certain foods and drinks can trigger or worsen acid reflux symptoms. If you suffer from acid reflux, it's best to avoid or limit the following foods and drinks:

- Spicy and fatty foods: Spicy foods can irritate the lining of the esophagus, while fatty foods can slow down the digestive process, leading to acid reflux symptoms. Examples include pizza, burgers, and fried foods.
- Citrus fruits and juices: Citrus fruits and juices, such as oranges, grapefruits, and lemons, can worsen acid reflux symptoms due to their high acidity levels.
- Tomatoes and tomato-based products: Tomatoes are highly acidic and can cause heartburn and acid

reflux symptoms. Avoid tomato-based products such as spaghetti sauce, ketchup, and tomato juice.

- Chocolate: Chocolate contains caffeine and theobromine, which can relax the lower esophageal sphincter (LES), the muscle that separates the stomach from the esophagus, allowing stomach acid to flow back up.
- Peppermint: Peppermint and peppermint oil can relax the LES and increase the risk of acid reflux symptoms.
- Alcohol: Alcohol can irritate the lining of the esophagus and increase the production of stomach acid, leading to acid reflux symptoms. Beer, wine, and spirits should be avoided or limited.
- Carbonated beverages: Carbonated beverages, such as soda and sparkling water, can increase the risk of acid reflux symptoms by putting pressure on the LES and forcing stomach acid back up into the esophagus.

Foods to Include

While some foods and drinks should be avoided, others can help alleviate the symptoms of acid reflux. The following are some of the best foods to include in a reflux-friendly diet:

- Non-citrus fruits: Non-citrus fruits, such as bananas, melons, and apples, are low in acidity and can help reduce acid reflux symptoms.
- Vegetables: Vegetables are low in fat and acidity and can help reduce the risk of acid reflux symptoms. Examples include broccoli, green

beans, and leafy greens.

- Lean protein: Lean protein sources, such as chicken, turkey, and fish, are low in fat and can help reduce the risk of acid reflux symptoms.
- Whole grains: Whole grains, such as brown rice, oatmeal, and whole-grain bread, are high in fiber and can help reduce the risk of acid reflux symptoms.
- Ginger: Ginger has anti-inflammatory properties and can help alleviate the symptoms of acid reflux. It can be added to meals or taken as a supplement.
- Alkaline water: Alkaline water can help neutralize stomach acid and reduce the risk of acid reflux symptoms. It can be purchased at health food stores or made at home by adding baking soda to water.
- Low-fat dairy: Low-fat dairy products, such as skim milk and yogurt, are low in fat and can help reduce the risk of acid reflux symptoms.

Other Tips for Managing Acid Reflux

In addition to making dietary changes, there are several other tips for managing acid reflux:

- Eat smaller, more frequent meals: Eating large meals can increase the risk of acid reflux symptoms. Instead, eat smaller, more frequent meals throughout the day to help reduce the risk.
- Avoid eating before bed: Eating before bed can increase the risk of acid reflux symptoms, so it's best to avoid eating for at least two to three hours before lying down.
- Elevate the head of your bed: Elevating the head

of your bed can help prevent stomach acid from flowing back up into the esophagus. Try using a wedge pillow or placing blocks under the head of your bed to elevate it.

- Avoid tight clothing: Tight clothing, especially around the waist, can put pressure on the stomach and increase the risk of acid reflux symptoms.
- Quit smoking: Smoking can increase the risk of acid reflux symptoms by relaxing the LES and increasing stomach acid production. Quitting smoking can help reduce the risk of acid reflux and improve overall health.
- Manage stress: Stress can increase the risk of acid reflux symptoms, so it's important to find ways to manage stress, such as practicing relaxation techniques or engaging in physical activity.

Acid reflux is a common condition that can cause discomfort and pain. While there are several medical treatments for acid reflux, making dietary changes can also help alleviate the symptoms. Avoiding certain foods and drinks and including others in a reflux-friendly diet can help reduce the risk of acid reflux symptoms. In addition, making lifestyle changes such as eating smaller, more frequent meals, avoiding eating before bed, and managing stress can also help reduce the risk of acid reflux. If you suffer from acid reflux, speak to your doctor or a registered dietitian to develop a personalized reflux-friendly diet plan that works for you.

Meal Planning For Acid Reflux:

Acid reflux, also known as gastroesophageal reflux disease (GERD), is a common digestive disorder that affects millions of people worldwide. The symptoms of acid reflux include heartburn, regurgitation, difficulty swallowing, chest pain, and other discomforts. The good news is that a well-planned diet can help reduce the frequency and severity of acid reflux symptoms. In this chapter, we will provide practical tips on how to plan meals that are conducive to reducing acid reflux symptoms. We will also provide sample meal plans for breakfast, lunch, and dinner.

Meal Planning for Acid Reflux

The key to planning meals for acid reflux is to avoid foods that can trigger symptoms. Common triggers include fatty foods, spicy foods, acidic foods, caffeine, alcohol, and carbonated beverages. You should also avoid eating large meals and lying down immediately after eating. Instead, aim to eat smaller, more frequent meals and wait at least 2-3 hours before lying down. Additionally, you should avoid eating within 2-3 hours of bedtime.

When planning meals for acid reflux, you should aim to include foods that are low in fat, low in acid, and easy to digest. Here are some practical tips to keep in mind:

- Choose lean proteins: Opt for lean proteins such as chicken, turkey, fish, and tofu instead of fatty meats like beef and pork. Be sure to prepare them without added fats or oils.
- Include complex carbohydrates: Choose whole grains such as brown rice, whole wheat pasta, and quinoa instead of refined carbohydrates like white bread and pasta.
- Add vegetables and fruits: Include a variety of vegetables and fruits in your meals. Opt for low-acid options such as broccoli, kale, spinach, sweet potatoes, bananas, melons, and berries.

- Avoid high-fat foods: Steer clear of high-fat foods like fried foods, cream-based sauces, and full-fat dairy products.
- Limit caffeine and alcohol: Both caffeine and alcohol can trigger acid reflux symptoms. Limit your intake of these beverages or avoid them altogether.
- Stay hydrated: Drink plenty of water throughout the day. Avoid drinking large amounts of fluids with meals, as this can cause stomach distension and contribute to acid reflux symptoms.

Sample Meal Plans

Now that we've covered the basics of meal planning for acid reflux, let's take a look at some sample meal plans for breakfast, lunch, and dinner.

Breakfast:

Option 1:

- 1 small bowl of oatmeal with sliced banana and almond milk
- 1 small apple
- 1 cup of green tea

Option 2:

- 2 scrambled eggs
- 1 slice of whole wheat toast
- 1 small orange
- 1 cup of herbal tea

Option 3:

- 1 cup of Greek yogurt with mixed berries
- 1 small whole wheat muffin
- 1 cup of decaf coffee

Lunch:

Option 1:

- Grilled chicken breast with steamed broccoli and brown rice
- 1 small apple
- Water or herbal tea

Option 2:

- Quinoa salad with mixed vegetables, avocado, and grilled shrimp
- 1 small orange
- Water or herbal tea

Option 3:

- Tofu stir-fry with mixed vegetables and brown rice
- 1 small banana
- Water or herbal tea

Dinner:

Option 1:

- Baked salmon with roasted sweet potatoes and green beans
- 1 small slice of whole wheat bread
- Water or herbal tea

Option 2:

- Whole wheat pasta with tomato sauce, grilled chicken, and mixed vegetables
- 1 small apple
- Water or herbal tea

Option 3:

- Grilled tofu with roasted vegetables and brown

rice
- 1 small orange
- Water or herbal tea

These meal plans are just a starting point. You can modify them to suit your tastes and preferences while still keeping in mind the principles of meal planning for acid reflux. Here are a few more tips to keep in mind when planning your meals:

- Don't skip meals: Skipping meals can cause your stomach to produce more acid, which can trigger acid reflux symptoms. Be sure to eat regular, small meals throughout the day.
- Keep a food diary: Keeping a food diary can help you identify which foods trigger your symptoms. Write down what you eat and how you feel afterwards to help you pinpoint any patterns.
- Eat slowly and mindfully: Eating slowly and mindfully can help reduce the amount of air you swallow, which can contribute to acid reflux symptoms. It can also help you enjoy your food more and feel more satisfied.
- Talk to your doctor: If you're experiencing frequent or severe acid reflux symptoms, talk to your doctor. They may be able to prescribe medication or recommend other treatments to help alleviate your symptoms.

In conclusion, planning meals for acid reflux can be challenging, but it's an important step in managing your symptoms. By avoiding trigger foods and including foods that are easy to digest, low in fat, and low in acid, you can reduce the frequency and severity of your symptoms. Use the sample meal plans above as a starting point, and don't be afraid to experiment with new recipes and ingredients. With a little creativity and planning, you can enjoy delicious, satisfying meals that are kind to your stomach.

Cooking Techniques For Acid Reflux:

Acid reflux, also known as gastroesophageal reflux disease (GERD), is a digestive disorder that causes stomach acid to flow back up into the esophagus, causing discomfort and inflammation. While there are various medications and lifestyle changes that can help manage GERD symptoms, dietary modifications can also play a significant role. In particular, cooking techniques that are gentle on the stomach can help reduce the risk of acid reflux and improve overall digestion. In this chapter, we'll explore some of the best cooking techniques for acid reflux.

Steaming

Steaming is a gentle cooking technique that involves cooking food over hot steam. Unlike boiling, which can cause food to become waterlogged and lose nutrients, steaming helps retain the natural flavors and nutrients of food while keeping it moist and tender. This makes steaming an excellent cooking method for those with acid reflux, as it avoids exposing food to harsh cooking oils and high temperatures that can trigger symptoms.

To steam food, you'll need a steamer basket or a steamer insert for a pot. Simply add water to the pot and bring it to a boil. Then, place the food in the steamer basket or insert and set it over the pot. Cover with a lid and allow the food to cook until tender. Steaming is ideal for cooking vegetables, fish, and chicken breasts, as well as grains such as rice and quinoa.

Poaching

Similar to steaming, poaching involves cooking food in liquid at a low temperature. This gentle cooking method is perfect for delicate foods such as eggs, fish, and chicken, as it keeps them moist and tender without adding additional fat or oils. Poaching can be done with water, broth, or wine, and can be seasoned with herbs and spices for added flavor.

To poach food, simply heat the liquid in a pot until it's hot but not boiling. Add the food to the pot and cook until tender. Poaching is a great cooking method for fish fillets, chicken breasts, and eggs.

Baking

While high-heat baking can cause food to become dry and tough, low-heat baking is a gentle cooking technique that can be beneficial for those with acid reflux. Baking allows food to cook slowly and evenly, resulting in tender and juicy meats, vegetables, and fruits. Additionally, baking can help retain the natural flavors and nutrients of food, making it a healthy and delicious cooking method.

To bake food, preheat the oven to the desired temperature and place the food in a baking dish. Cover with foil and bake until tender. Baking is ideal for chicken breasts, fish fillets, vegetables, and fruits.

Grilling

While grilling is generally not recommended for those with acid reflux, there are ways to make this cooking method more stomach-friendly. First, avoid using high-fat meats and marinades that can trigger symptoms. Instead, opt for lean meats such as chicken or fish, and season with herbs and spices rather than acidic ingredients such as lemon juice or vinegar. Additionally, grilling fruits and vegetables can be a healthy and delicious way to incorporate more plant-based foods into your diet.

To grill food, preheat the grill to the desired temperature and brush the grates with oil to prevent sticking. Add the food to the grill and cook until tender, flipping halfway through. Grilling is ideal for chicken breasts, fish fillets, and vegetables such as zucchini, peppers, and mushrooms.

Stir-Frying

Stir-frying is a quick and easy cooking technique that involves cooking food in a small amount of oil over high heat. This cooking method can be beneficial for those with acid reflux, as it allows food to cook quickly and retain its natural flavors and nutrients. Additionally, stir-frying can help reduce the need for added salt and other high-fat ingredients, making it a healthy and flavorful option.

To stir-fry, heat a small amount of oil in a wok or large skillet over high heat. Add the food and cook, stirring frequently, until tender. Stir-frying is ideal for vegetables, lean proteins such as chicken and shrimp, and grains such as rice and quinoa.

Slow Cooking

Slow cooking is a gentle cooking method that involves cooking food over low heat for an extended period of time. This cooking technique is ideal for tough cuts of meat, as it allows them to become tender and juicy without exposing them to high temperatures. Additionally, slow cooking can help retain the natural flavors and nutrients of food, making it a healthy and delicious option for those with acid reflux.

To slow cook food, place it in a slow cooker or Dutch oven with a small amount of liquid. Cover and cook on low heat for several hours, until the food is tender. Slow cooking is ideal for beef roasts, pork shoulder, and stews.

Blending

Blending is a cooking technique that involves pureeing food in a blender or food processor. This cooking method can be beneficial for those with acid reflux, as it allows food to become more easily digestible and reduces the risk of irritation. Additionally, blending can help retain the natural flavors and nutrients of food, making it a healthy and delicious option for smoothies, soups, and sauces.

To blend food, simply add it to a blender or food processor and blend until smooth. Blending is ideal for smoothies, soups, and sauces.

In addition to these cooking techniques, there are a few other tips that can help reduce the risk of acid reflux during mealtime. First, it's important to avoid high-fat and fried foods, as they can trigger symptoms. Instead, opt for lean proteins, vegetables, and fruits. Additionally, it's important to eat slowly and chew food thoroughly to aid digestion. Finally, avoid eating large meals before bedtime, as this can increase the risk of acid reflux.

In conclusion, there are several cooking techniques that can be beneficial for those with acid reflux. Steaming, poaching, baking, grilling, stir-frying, slow cooking, and blending are all gentle cooking methods that can help reduce the risk of irritation and improve overall digestion. By incorporating these cooking techniques into your meal planning, you can enjoy delicious and healthy meals that are gentle on the stomach.

Eating Out with Acid Reflux:

Eating out can be challenging for those with acid reflux, as many restaurant foods can trigger symptoms. However, with a little planning and knowledge, it is possible to enjoy dining out while still managing acid reflux symptoms. In this chapter, we will provide practical tips for eating out with acid reflux, including how to choose reflux-friendly options and what to avoid.

Research the Restaurant

Before dining out, it's a good idea to research the restaurant's menu and reviews to get a sense of the types of foods they offer. Look for restaurants that offer a variety of healthy options, such as salads, lean proteins, and grilled or steamed vegetables. Additionally, read reviews to see if other diners with acid reflux have had positive experiences at the restaurant.

Ask Questions

When dining out, don't be afraid to ask your server about the ingredients and preparation methods of certain dishes. Ask if a dish can be prepared without high-fat ingredients, such as butter or cream, and if it can be cooked without added salt or spices. Additionally, ask if the restaurant offers any reflux-friendly options or substitutions.

Choose Reflux-Friendly Options

When choosing a meal, look for options that are low in fat and spices. Opt for grilled or steamed proteins, such as chicken or fish, and choose dishes that are served with vegetables or a side salad. Avoid dishes that are deep-fried or smothered in sauces or gravy, as they can trigger symptoms. Additionally, choose whole-grain options, such as brown rice or whole-wheat pasta, instead of refined grains, which can be more irritating.

Avoid Trigger Foods

Certain foods are known to trigger acid reflux symptoms, such as spicy foods, citrus fruits, and tomatoes. It's important to avoid these trigger foods when dining out to prevent symptoms. Additionally, avoid alcohol and carbonated beverages, as they can increase the risk of reflux.

Eat Smaller Meals

When dining out, it's easy to overindulge and eat larger portions than you would at home. However, eating large meals can increase the risk of acid reflux symptoms. Instead, opt for smaller, more frequent meals throughout the day. Consider ordering an appetizer or splitting an entrée with a dining partner to reduce portion sizes.

Take Your Time

Eating slowly and chewing food thoroughly can help aid digestion and reduce the risk of acid reflux symptoms. Take your time when dining out, and savor each bite. Additionally, avoid rushing through your meal, as this can increase the risk of swallowing air, which can trigger symptoms.

Bring Your Own Condiments

Many condiments, such as ketchup and mustard, can be high in acid and trigger symptoms. Consider bringing your own reflux-friendly condiments, such as honey or low-acid hot sauce, to use when dining out. Additionally, ask for dressings and sauces on the side, so you can control the amount you consume.

Stay Upright After Eating

After finishing your meal, avoid lying down or reclining for at least 2-3 hours to prevent acid reflux symptoms. Instead, stay upright and take a leisurely walk or engage in light activity to aid digestion.

In conclusion, eating out with acid reflux can be challenging, but with a little planning and knowledge, it is possible to enjoy dining out while still managing symptoms. Researching the restaurant's menu, asking questions, choosing reflux-friendly options, avoiding trigger foods, eating smaller meals, taking your time, bringing your own condiments, and staying upright after eating can all help reduce the risk of acid reflux symptoms when dining out. By incorporating these tips into your dining out routine, you can enjoy delicious and healthy meals without sacrificing your acid reflux management.

It's important to remember that everyone's triggers and symptoms may differ, so it's essential to listen to your body and make choices that work for you. Keeping a food diary and noting any symptoms can help identify trigger foods and guide your choices when dining out.

Additionally, it's important to communicate your needs with your dining companions and the restaurant staff. Don't be afraid to speak up and let them know about your dietary restrictions and preferences. Many restaurants are willing to accommodate special requests, so don't hesitate to ask.

Lastly, if you're unsure about a particular dish or restaurant, it's always better to err on the side of caution and choose a simpler, more straightforward meal. Remember, your health and well-being are the most important things, and it's better to miss out on a particular dish than to suffer from uncomfortable symptoms.

In summary, eating out with acid reflux can be challenging, but with a little planning and knowledge, it's possible to enjoy dining out while still managing symptoms. By researching the restaurant, asking questions, choosing reflux-friendly options, avoiding trigger foods, eating smaller meals, taking your time, bringing your own condiments, and staying upright after eating, you can reduce the risk of acid reflux symptoms when dining out. Remember to communicate your needs with your dining companions and the restaurant staff and listen to your body to make choices that work for you. With these tips, you can confidently navigate the dining out world while managing your acid reflux symptoms.

Conclusion And Final Thoughts:

In conclusion, living with acid reflux can be challenging, but it's possible to manage symptoms and improve quality of life through dietary changes and lifestyle modifications. By avoiding trigger foods, eating smaller meals, chewing food thoroughly, staying upright after eating, and incorporating reflux-friendly ingredients and cooking techniques, it's possible to reduce the risk of acid reflux symptoms and enjoy a varied and satisfying diet.

It's important to remember that everyone's triggers and symptoms may differ, so it's essential to listen to your body and make choices that work for you. Keeping a food diary and noting any symptoms can help identify trigger foods and guide your choices.

In addition to dietary changes, lifestyle modifications can also help manage acid reflux symptoms. This includes avoiding tight clothing, elevating the head of the bed, quitting smoking, and reducing stress.

It's also important to maintain a healthy weight, as excess weight can contribute to acid reflux symptoms. Regular exercise, stress management techniques, and adequate sleep can all contribute to maintaining a healthy weight and reducing the risk of acid reflux symptoms.

Remember that it's important to work with a healthcare professional to manage your acid reflux symptoms, as they can provide guidance on the best course of treatment and any necessary medication.

In terms of continuing to follow a reflux-friendly diet, it's important to approach it as a lifestyle change rather than a temporary fix. This means finding recipes and ingredients that you enjoy, incorporating variety and balance into your meals, and focusing on the positive aspects of the diet rather than feeling restricted.

It can also be helpful to find a support system, whether that's through friends and family, online communities, or support groups. Sharing your experiences and tips with others can provide motivation and encouragement to continue following a reflux-friendly diet.

Lastly, don't be too hard on yourself if you slip up or have a meal that triggers symptoms. Remember that managing acid reflux is a journey, and it's important to be kind and patient with yourself along the way.

In summary, living with acid reflux requires dietary and lifestyle changes, but it's possible to manage symptoms and enjoy a varied and satisfying diet. By avoiding trigger foods, incorporating reflux-friendly ingredients and cooking techniques, and making lifestyle modifications, it's possible to reduce the risk of acid reflux symptoms and improve quality of life. Remember to approach the diet as a lifestyle change, find a support system, and be patient and kind to yourself along the way. With these tips and a positive mindset, you can continue to thrive while managing your acid reflux symptoms.

CHAPTER TWO

Oatmeal with Banana and Honey
Ingredients:

- 1/2 cup rolled oats
- 1 cup water or milk
- 1/2 banana, sliced
- 1 tsp honey

Instructions:

- In a small saucepan, bring the water or milk to a boil.
- Add the rolled oats and stir.
- Reduce the heat to low and simmer for 5-7 minutes, stirring occasionally.
- Once the oatmeal is cooked to your liking, remove from heat and let cool for a minute.
- Top with sliced banana and drizzle with honey. Serve immediately.

Avocado Toast with Turkey Bacon
Ingredients:

- 1 slice of whole-grain bread
- 1/2 ripe avocado, mashed
- 2 slices of turkey bacon, cooked
- Salt and pepper to taste

Instructions:

- Toast the bread until golden brown.
- While the bread is toasting, cook the turkey bacon

in a non-stick pan until crispy.
- Spread the mashed avocado on the toasted bread.
- Top with the cooked turkey bacon slices.
- Sprinkle with salt and pepper to taste. Serve immediately.

Greek Yogurt Parfait
Ingredients:

- 1 cup Greek yogurt
- 1/2 cup granola
- 1/2 cup mixed berries (e.g. strawberries, blueberries, raspberries)
- 1 tsp honey

Instructions:

- In a bowl or jar, layer Greek yogurt, granola, and mixed berries.
- Drizzle with honey.
- Repeat layering until you have used up all of the ingredients.
- Serve immediately or refrigerate for later.

Veggie Omelet
Ingredients:

- 2 eggs
- 1 tbsp milk
- 1/4 cup chopped vegetables (e.g. spinach, mushrooms, bell peppers)
- Salt and pepper to taste
- 1 tsp olive oil

Instructions:

- In a small bowl, whisk together eggs and milk.
- Heat olive oil in a non-stick pan over medium heat.
- Add chopped vegetables and sauté until tender.
- Pour the egg mixture into the pan and let cook for 2-3 minutes or until the bottom is set.
- Use a spatula to flip the omelet and cook for another 1-2 minutes on the other side.
- Season with salt and pepper to taste. Serve immediately.

Chicken and Rice Soup

Ingredients:

- 1 chicken breast, cooked and shredded
- 1/2 cup cooked white rice
- 2 cups low-sodium chicken broth
- 1/2 cup chopped carrots
- 1/2 cup chopped celery
- Salt and pepper to taste

Instructions:

- In a pot, bring the chicken broth to a boil.
- Add the chopped carrots and celery and simmer for 5-7 minutes.
- Add the cooked chicken and cooked rice and simmer for another 5-7 minutes.
- Season with salt and pepper to taste. Serve hot.

Tuna Salad with Avocado Dressing

Ingredients:

- 1 can of tuna, drained
- 1/4 cup diced celery

- 1/4 cup diced red onion
- 2 tbsp plain Greek yogurt
- 1 tbsp lemon juice
- Salt and pepper to taste
- 1/2 avocado, mashed

Instructions:

- In a bowl, mix together tuna, celery, and red onion.
- In a separate bowl, whisk together Greek yogurt, lemon juice, and salt and pepper.
- Pour the dressing over the tuna mixture and stir until combined.
- Spread the mashed avocado on a plate and top with the tuna salad. Serve cold.

Veggie and Quinoa Salad

Ingredients:

- 1/2 cup cooked quinoa
- 1/2 cup chopped cucumber
- 1/2 cup chopped bell peppers
- 1/4 cup chopped red onion
- 2 tbsp olive oil
- 2 tbsp balsamic vinegar
- Salt and pepper to taste

Instructions:

- In a bowl, mix together cooked quinoa, chopped cucumber, chopped bell peppers, and chopped red onion.
- In a separate bowl, whisk together olive oil, balsamic vinegar, and salt and pepper.
- Pour the dressing over the quinoa mixture and stir

until combined.
- Serve cold.

Grilled Chicken Sandwich
Ingredients:

- 1 chicken breast, grilled and sliced
- 2 slices of whole-grain bread
- 1/4 avocado, sliced
- 1 tbsp hummus
- 1 tbsp Dijon mustard
- Salt and pepper to taste

Instructions:

- Toast the bread until golden brown.
- Spread hummus on one side of the bread and Dijon mustard on the other.
- Layer sliced avocado and grilled chicken on one slice of bread.
- Sprinkle with salt and pepper to taste.
- Top with the other slice of bread. Serve hot.

Tomato and Basil Soup
Ingredients:

- 4 ripe tomatoes, chopped
- 1/4 cup chopped onion
- 2 cups low-sodium chicken broth
- 2 tbsp olive oil
- 1/4 cup chopped fresh basil
- Salt and pepper to taste

Instructions:

- In a pot, heat olive oil over medium heat.

- Add chopped onion and sauté for 2-3 minutes.
- Add chopped tomatoes and sauté for another 2-3 minutes.
- Add chicken broth and bring to a boil.
- Reduce heat and simmer for 10-15 minutes.
- Add chopped fresh basil and season with salt and pepper to taste.
- Use an immersion blender to blend the soup until smooth.
- Serve hot.

Turkey and Avocado Wrap

Ingredients:

- 1 whole-grain tortilla
- 2 oz sliced turkey breast
- 1/4 avocado, sliced
- 1/4 cup chopped romaine lettuce
- 2 tbsp plain Greek yogurt
- Salt and pepper to taste

Instructions:

- Lay the tortilla flat on a plate.
- Spread Greek yogurt on the tortilla.
- Layer sliced turkey, sliced avocado, and chopped romaine lettuce on top of the Greek yogurt.
- Sprinkle with salt and pepper to taste.
- Roll up the tortilla tightly and serve cold.

Chickpea and Spinach Salad

Ingredients:

- 1 can of chickpeas, drained and rinsed
- 2 cups fresh baby spinach

- 1/2 cup chopped cucumber
- 1/4 cup chopped red onion
- 2 tbsp olive oil
- 2 tbsp lemon juice
- Salt and pepper to taste

Instructions:

- In a bowl, mix together chickpeas, baby spinach, chopped cucumber, and chopped red onion.
- In a separate bowl, whisk together olive oil, lemon juice, and salt and pepper.
- Pour the dressing over the salad mixture and toss until combined.
- Serve cold.

Baked Salmon with Roasted Vegetables
Ingredients:

- 4 salmon fillets
- 1 zucchini, sliced
- 1 red bell pepper, sliced
- 1 yellow onion, sliced
- 2 tbsp olive oil
- Salt and pepper to taste

Instructions:

- Preheat the oven to 375°F.
- Place the salmon fillets on a baking sheet lined with parchment paper.
- In a bowl, toss the sliced zucchini, red bell pepper, and yellow onion with olive oil, salt, and pepper.
- Spread the vegetables on the baking sheet around the salmon fillets.
- Bake for 15-20 minutes or until the salmon is

cooked through and the vegetables are tender.

Chicken and Vegetable Stir-Fry

Ingredients:

- 2 boneless, skinless chicken breasts, sliced
- 1 cup broccoli florets
- 1 cup sliced carrots
- 1 cup sliced bell peppers
- 1 tbsp olive oil
- 2 cloves garlic, minced
- Salt and pepper to taste

Instructions:

- Heat the olive oil in a large skillet over medium-high heat.
- Add the chicken and cook until browned and cooked through, about 5-7 minutes.
- Add the broccoli florets, sliced carrots, and sliced bell peppers to the skillet.
- Add minced garlic, salt, and pepper to taste.
- Stir-fry until the vegetables are tender, about 5-7 minutes.

Quinoa Stuffed Peppers

Ingredients:

- 4 bell peppers, tops cut off and seeded
- 1 cup quinoa, rinsed
- 1 can black beans, drained and rinsed
- 1 cup diced tomatoes
- 1 cup chopped spinach
- 1 tsp cumin
- 1 tsp chili powder

- Salt and pepper to taste

Instructions:

- Preheat the oven to 375°F.
- In a large bowl, mix together the quinoa, black beans, diced tomatoes, chopped spinach, cumin, chili powder, salt, and pepper.
- Spoon the quinoa mixture into the bell peppers.
- Place the stuffed bell peppers in a baking dish and bake for 30-40 minutes or until the peppers are tender and the filling is heated through.

Baked Sweet Potato with Black Bean Chili

Ingredients:

- 4 small sweet potatoes
- 1 can black beans, drained and rinsed
- 1 can diced tomatoes
- 1 tbsp olive oil
- 1 tbsp chili powder
- 1 tsp cumin
- Salt and pepper to taste

Instructions:

- Preheat the oven to 375°F.
- Pierce the sweet potatoes with a fork several times.
- Place the sweet potatoes on a baking sheet lined with parchment paper and bake for 45-60 minutes or until tender.
- In a skillet, heat the olive oil over medium-high heat.
- Add the black beans, diced tomatoes, chili powder, cumin, salt, and pepper.

- Cook for 10-15 minutes or until heated through.
- Serve the baked sweet potatoes topped with the black bean chili.

Lentil Soup

Ingredients:

- 1 cup dried lentils
- 1 onion, chopped
- 2 cloves garlic, minced
- 2 carrots, peeled and chopped
- 2 celery stalks, chopped
- 4 cups low-sodium chicken or vegetable broth
- 1 tsp dried thyme
- Salt and pepper to taste

Instructions

- Rinse the lentils and set them aside.
- In a large pot, heat some oil over medium-high heat. Add the chopped onion and sauté until translucent, about 5-7 minutes.
- Add the minced garlic and sauté for another minute.
- Add the chopped carrots and celery to the pot and sauté for another 5-7 minutes.
- Add the lentils, broth, dried thyme, salt, and pepper to the pot. Bring to a boil, then reduce the heat and simmer for 30-40 minutes or until the lentils are tender.
- Serve hot.

Grilled Chicken with Roasted Vegetables

Ingredients:

- 2 boneless, skinless chicken breasts
- 1 zucchini, sliced
- 1 yellow squash, sliced
- 1 red onion, sliced
- 2 tbsp olive oil
- Salt and pepper to taste

Instructions:

- Preheat a grill or grill pan over medium-high heat.
- Season the chicken breasts with salt and pepper.
- Grill the chicken for 5-6 minutes per side or until cooked through.
- In a bowl, toss the sliced zucchini, yellow squash, and red onion with olive oil, salt, and pepper.
- Spread the vegetables on a baking sheet and roast in the oven at 375°F for 15-20 minutes or until tender.
- Serve the grilled chicken with the roasted vegetables.

Spinach and Mushroom Frittata

Ingredients:

- 6 large eggs
- 1/4 cup low-fat milk
- 1 cup chopped spinach
- 1 cup sliced mushrooms
- 1/2 onion, chopped
- 1 tbsp olive oil
- Salt and pepper to taste

Instructions:

- Preheat the oven to 375°F.
- In a skillet, heat the olive oil over medium-high

heat.
- Add the chopped onion and sauté until translucent, about 5-7 minutes.
- Add the sliced mushrooms and sauté for another 5-7 minutes or until tender.
- Add the chopped spinach to the skillet and sauté until wilted.
- In a bowl, whisk together the eggs, low-fat milk, salt, and pepper.
- Pour the egg mixture over the vegetables in the skillet.
- Transfer the skillet to the oven and bake for 15-20 minutes or until the frittata is set and golden brown.
- Slice and serve.

Baked Sweet Potato Chips
Ingredients:

- 1 sweet potato, sliced thinly
- 1 tbsp olive oil
- Salt and pepper to taste

Instructions:

- Preheat the oven to 375°F.
- Toss the sweet potato slices with olive oil, salt, and pepper in a bowl.
- Spread the sweet potato slices on a baking sheet.
- Bake for 15-20 minutes or until crispy.
- Serve and enjoy.

Yogurt and Berry Parfait
Ingredients:

- 1 cup plain low-fat yogurt
- 1/2 cup mixed berries (such as blueberries, raspberries, and strawberries)
- 1/4 cup granola
- 1 tsp honey (optional)

Instructions:

- In a bowl, layer the yogurt, mixed berries, and granola.
- Drizzle honey on top, if desired.
- Serve and enjoy.

Hummus and Vegetable Plate
Ingredients:

- 1/2 cup hummus
- Carrot sticks
- Cucumber slices
- Bell pepper slices

Instructions:

- Arrange the hummus and vegetable slices on a plate.
- Serve and enjoy.

Rice Cake with Almond Butter and Banana
Ingredients:

- 1 rice cake
- 1 tbsp almond butter
- 1/2 banana, sliced

Instructions:

- Spread the almond butter on the rice cake.
- Top with sliced banana.

- Serve and enjoy.

Apple Slices with Peanut Butter

Ingredients:

- 1 apple, sliced
- 2 tbsp peanut butter

Instructions:

- Spread peanut butter on the apple slices.
- Serve and enjoy.

Trail Mix

Ingredients:

- 1/2 cup mixed nuts (such as almonds, cashews, and walnuts)
- 1/4 cup dried fruit (such as raisins or cranberries)
- 1/4 cup whole-grain cereal

Instructions:

- Mix together the nuts, dried fruit, and whole-grain cereal in a bowl.
- Serve and enjoy.

Roasted Chickpeas

Ingredients:

- 1 can chickpeas, rinsed and drained
- 1 tbsp olive oil
- 1/2 tsp garlic powder
- 1/2 tsp cumin
- 1/4 tsp paprika
- Salt and pepper to taste

Instructions:

- Preheat the oven to 375°F.
- Toss the chickpeas with olive oil, garlic powder, cumin, paprika, salt, and pepper in a bowl.
- Spread the chickpeas on a baking sheet.
- Bake for 25-30 minutes or until crispy.
- Serve and enjoy.

Ginger Tea

Ingredients:

- 1 inch piece of ginger root, sliced
- 2 cups of water
- Honey or lemon (optional)

Instructions:

- Boil the sliced ginger root in 2 cups of water for 10 minutes.
- Strain the ginger tea into a cup.
- Add honey or lemon, if desired.
- Serve and enjoy.

Green Smoothie

Ingredients:

- 1 cup spinach
- 1/2 banana
- 1/2 cup pineapple chunks
- 1/2 cup almond milk

Instructions:

- Add all the ingredients to a blender and blend until smooth.
- Serve and enjoy.

Turmeric Milk

Ingredients:

- 1 cup unsweetened almond milk
- 1/2 tsp ground turmeric
- 1/2 tsp ground cinnamon
- 1/2 tsp honey

Instructions:

- Heat the almond milk in a small saucepan over medium heat.
- Add turmeric, cinnamon, and honey and stir until well combined.
- Heat the mixture until it reaches a simmer.
- Remove from heat and let cool for a few minutes.
- Serve and enjoy.

Banana Oatmeal Smoothie

Ingredients:

- 1 ripe banana
- 1/2 cup rolled oats
- 1 cup unsweetened almond milk
- 1/2 tsp vanilla extract
- 1 tsp honey (optional)

Instructions:

- Add all the ingredients to a blender and blend until smooth.
- Serve and enjoy.

Iced Chamomile Tea

Ingredients:

- 2 chamomile tea bags
- 2 cups of water
- 1/2 cup ice cubes
- Honey or lemon (optional)

Instructions:

- Boil the water and steep the tea bags for 5-10 minutes.
- Remove the tea bags and let the tea cool.
- Add ice cubes to a glass and pour the tea over them.
- Add honey or lemon, if desired.
- Serve and enjoy.

Carrot and Ginger Smoothie

Ingredients:

- 1 carrot, peeled and chopped
- 1 inch piece of ginger root, peeled and chopped
- 1/2 cup pineapple chunks
- 1/2 cup unsweetened almond milk

Instructions:

- Add all the ingredients to a blender and blend until smooth.
- Serve and enjoy.

Hot Chocolate

Ingredients:

- 1 cup unsweetened almond milk
- 1 tbsp unsweetened cocoa powder
- 1/2 tsp vanilla extract
- 1 tsp honey (optional)

Instructions:

- Heat the almond milk in a small saucepan over medium heat.
- Add cocoa powder, vanilla extract, and honey and stir until well combined.
- Heat the mixture until it reaches a simmer.
- Remove from heat and let cool for a few minutes.
- Serve and enjoy.

Baked Apples

Ingredients:

- 4 apples
- 2 tbsp honey
- 1/2 tsp cinnamon
- 1/4 cup chopped nuts (optional)

Instructions:

- Preheat the oven to 350°F (180°C).
- Cut the top off each apple and remove the core and seeds.
- Mix the honey and cinnamon in a small bowl and brush the mixture inside each apple.
- Place the apples in a baking dish and sprinkle with chopped nuts (optional).
- Bake for 25-30 minutes or until the apples are tender.
- Serve warm and enjoy.

Banana Ice Cream

Ingredients:

- 2 ripe bananas, sliced and frozen
- 1/2 cup unsweetened almond milk

- 1 tsp vanilla extract

Instructions:

- Add the frozen bananas, almond milk, and vanilla extract to a blender.
- Blend until smooth and creamy.
- Serve immediately and enjoy.

Avocado Chocolate Mousse
Ingredients:

- 2 ripe avocados
- 1/4 cup unsweetened cocoa powder
- 1/4 cup honey
- 1 tsp vanilla extract

Instructions:

- Cut the avocados in half, remove the pit and scoop out the flesh.
- Add the avocado, cocoa powder, honey, and vanilla extract to a blender.
- Blend until smooth and creamy.
- Chill the mousse in the refrigerator for at least 30 minutes.
- Serve and enjoy.

Coconut Rice Pudding
Ingredients:

- 1 cup cooked white rice
- 1 can coconut milk
- 1/4 cup honey
- 1/2 tsp vanilla extract
- 1/4 tsp ground cinnamon

Instructions:

- In a saucepan, heat the cooked rice and coconut milk over medium heat.
- Add honey, vanilla extract, and cinnamon and stir until well combined.
- Cook for 10-15 minutes, stirring occasionally until the mixture thickens.
- Remove from heat and let cool.
- Serve and enjoy.

Baked Pears with Almond Crumble

Ingredients:

- 4 pears, peeled and cored
- 1/2 cup almond flour
- 1/4 cup rolled oats
- 1/4 cup chopped almonds
- 2 tbsp honey
- 1/2 tsp cinnamon
- 1/4 tsp salt
- 2 tbsp coconut oil, melted

Instructions:

- Preheat the oven to 375°F (190°C).
- Place the pears in a baking dish.
- In a small bowl, mix the almond flour, oats, chopped almonds, honey, cinnamon, salt, and melted coconut oil until well combined.
- Spoon the crumble mixture over the pears.
- Bake for 25-30 minutes or until the pears are tender and the crumble is golden brown.
- Serve warm and enjoy.

Sweet Potato Pie

Ingredients:

- 1 1/2 cups cooked sweet potato, mashed
- 1/2 cup unsweetened almond milk
- 1/4 cup honey
- 1/2 tsp ground cinnamon
- 1/4 tsp ground ginger
- 1/4 tsp ground nutmeg
- 2 eggs
- 1 pie crust

Instructions:

- Preheat the oven to 350°F (180°C).
- In a large bowl, mix the mashed sweet potato, almond milk, honey, cinnamon, ginger, nutmeg, and eggs until well combined.
- Pour the mixture into the pie crust.
- Bake for 45-50 minutes or until the filling is set and the crust is golden brown.
- 5. Let cool for 10-15 minutes before slicing and serving.

Yogurt Parfait with Berries and Granola

Ingredients:

- 1 cup plain Greek yogurt
- 1/2 cup fresh berries (such as blueberries, strawberries, or raspberries)
- 1/4 cup low-acid granola
- 1 tbsp honey

Instructions:

- In a small bowl, mix the Greek yogurt and honey

until well combined.
- Layer the yogurt mixture, berries, and granola in a glass or jar.
- Repeat layers until all ingredients are used up.
- Serve and enjoy.

CONCLUSION

In "The Acid Reflux Cookbook," we've explored the impact of diet on acid reflux and provided a range of delicious and reflux-friendly recipes to help manage symptoms. We've learned about the foods and ingredients that can trigger acid reflux, as well as those that can help soothe and prevent symptoms. And we've explored cooking techniques and dining out tips that can make living with acid reflux more manageable and enjoyable.

We hope that this cookbook has been a valuable resource for you, whether you've been managing acid reflux for years or are just starting to explore dietary changes. By making simple yet effective changes to your diet and lifestyle, you can manage your symptoms and live a happier and healthier life.

Remember, living with acid reflux doesn't mean sacrificing flavor and variety in your diet. In fact, with the recipes in this cookbook, you'll discover a world of delicious and reflux-friendly options that you may not have tried before. From savory soups to sweet desserts, and everything in between, you'll find something for every meal and every occasion.

But managing acid reflux is not just about the food you eat. It's also about making healthy lifestyle choices, such as exercising regularly, getting enough sleep, and reducing stress. By taking care of your overall health, you'll not only manage your acid reflux symptoms, but you'll also improve your quality of life.

We hope that the resources provided in this cookbook, including information on different types of acid reflux and stress management techniques, have been helpful in your journey towards better health. And we encourage you to continue exploring new and delicious ways to manage your acid reflux symptoms.

Thank you for choosing "The Acid Reflux Cookbook" as your guide to living deliciously with acid reflux. We wish you all the best in your journey towards better health and happiness.